Contents

Welcome!

Welcome to the 7 minute workout, a revolutionary exercise plan to help anyone burn fat, beat stress and create lean muscle. Whether you're an entrepreneur, a busy mum or you simply spend long hours sitting behind a desk and commuting to work it is becoming increasingly difficult to fit a healthy lifestyle around other commitments. Being healthy is a choice and time is a commodity we are very short of in this day and age, so we choose to neglect exercise and healthy eating in favour of lazier options that don't interfere with our already hectic schedules.

My name is Kelly and I have been a personal trainer for over 10 years and an avid sportswomen my whole life. You may think it's easy for me as exercise is my job, however I know as well as anyone that fitting my own workouts around my business, my family and my friends takes planning and commitment. After a 10 hour day I don't always feel like going out for a run or getting myself down to the gym, but yes as a trainer I do have an advantage.

After 10 years of listening to my client's wants and needs it's become increasingly clear that people need exercise to fit in with them, not the other way around. I have trained people from all walks of life including full time Models, TV presenters, CEO's, TV stars and stay at home Mums. I have worked with teachers, Doctors, journalists, business consultants and recruitment specialists and being located on the edge of London most of my clients commute on a daily basis. Their days start at 5:30am and finish at 7pm when they travel home to feed their children, see their partners and get ready to do it all again. There is simply not time for an hour in the gym.

But wait…. Do we really need an hour in the gym? In short… No. What we do need is an efficient method of working the body to burn as many calories as we can in the shortest possible time frame. We need routines that work the body from every angle to create shape and definition. We need to know how to wake up the muscles to keep them firing throughout the day and how to utilise our energy even at rest. And we can do that in less than 10 minutes.

7 Minutes to get the body of your dreams

So why 7 minutes?

It's important to exercise and move every day to keep your metabolism active. A sedentary lifestyle creates sluggish hormones which slow down all the normal chemical processes including fat burning.

You may think you do not have time to exercise but even just 7 Minutes a day can maintain and even change your body shape and simply keep a natural healthy balance.

We have a resting metabolic rate (basal metabolic rate) which is the amount of calories we need at rest, which for the average women is 1300 calories. Any food is converted to glycogen in the liver and stored in the muscles. Once we have reached the basal level any other calories will be stored in the fat cells.

When we exercise we convert the glycogen in our muscles into heat and water through chemical reactions and once we deplete those glycogen stores we start to burn fat as a fuel.

Most people will spend an average of 40 minutes on a gym machine such as the treadmill never really pushing themselves over the mythical 'fat burning zone'. They will then use the next 20 minutes to aimlessly thrash out 15 reps on each of the weights machines without really ever activating the right muscles. By the time they finish their workout their muscles have adapted to the pace and their metabolism will have stabilised never having depleted the glycogen stores in the muscle and therefore barely touching the fat cells. They will burn calories but this will effectively stop once they leave the gym and will quickly return to their resting rate. It's a very slow process.

So let's save some time. Let's compress a workout into 7 minutes and focus on exercises that work the whole body, through all 3 planes of motion to manipulate the fat burning system into burning lots more calories at rest.

To reach this level our body has to overcome its anaerobic threshold meaning we are working at a speed beyond which our lungs can comfortably supply oxygen. We end up working without oxygen thus fatiguing very quickly. With this in mind it is virtually impossible to continue a HIIT workout for longer than 30 minutes, after this time we cannot continue at the same pace or intensity and the workout loses it value. We only want to work out for 7 minutes so we have the ability to really push the limits.

When we force the body to work out of its comfort zone in this way we increase the lactic acid levels in the blood stream (as the body can only push through these lactic acid levels so far, the workouts will have to be short) which has a positive impact on the release of fat burning hormones. Working above the lactic threshold will increase Growth hormone production to rebuild and repair the muscles helping to preserve lean muscle mass. This in turn stimulates the release of the hormones Adiponectin and PGC1 from fatty tissues, both of which kick start metabolic reactions and break down body fat.

The increase of these hormones helps to counter the effects of cortisol on the body. Cortisol is a stress hormone which is released as a response to high levels of physical and mental stress, to help stabilise and maintain blood sugar levels. Constant high levels in the blood stream however can have an inflammatory effect, inhibiting body fat and breaking down lean muscle mass. To put this in perspective, Cortisol is found to be highest in endurance athletes who are renowned for having very low muscle mass.

Long periods of aerobic exercise (for example 40 minutes on a cross trainer at the same pace) will produce high levels of cortisol and over a long period this will equate to a lower metabolism and softer muscle tissue. This makes burning fat harder and is often the reason very active and slim people will end up with soft rolls of body fat on the abdomen.

How can 7 minutes be effective?

We need to review the types of exercises we use in our workouts to get the most effective results. Each workout needs to use big and small muscle groups all at the same time. The more muscles we use in one go the more calories we need and effectually burn. To achieve this each exercise needs to be high in intensity, impact and work across the muscle groups. By this I mean one directional movements such as bicep curls have no place in this plan but multidirectional moves i.e. combat press ups that engage the biceps, triceps, core, shoulders and gluts are featured heavily. Each move needs to be explosive performed as quickly as possible with lots of force and power. As its only 7 minutes there is no reason to pace yourself so push hard from the beginning to get the best results.

Waking up the core

As we work through the program you will start to notice the absence of sit ups and crunches, two of the favoured exercises amongst gym goers. Now while I feel there is a place for both in certain circumstances, I firmly believe that no amount of crunches or sit ups will give you a six pack and they most definitely will not burn fat unless we do lots and lots of them. As we only have 7 minutes to kick start the fat burning machine we will not be using them. Instead, we are going to focus on waking up the 'core' a collection of muscles including the rectus abdominals (the six pack), the transverse abdominals, the internal and external oblique's, spinal erectors and the multifidus. We also use the hip flexors a collection of muscles across the top of the thigh which literally 'flex' the hip.

An abdominal crunch requires a lift from a lying position all the way to sitting. We use very few abdominal muscles to do this but a lot of strain is placed on the hip flexors, a collection of muscles that literally 'flex' the hip. During a sit up the hip flexors pull on the lower back tipping the pelvis forwards and pushing the internal organs against the abdomen creating in effect a 'pot belly' look. Far from flattening the stomach, all we actually achieve is a tight lower back and a weak posture.

To fully activate the core we need to use all the core muscles at once. This again involves big movements such as planks; burpee's, jumps and twists. It's also important to burn the fat on top. Many people already have strong defined abdominals but they are sitting under a layer of fat. Fortunately the exercises we will cover in this workout burn fat as well as tone the muscle.

Muscle Awareness

Throughout each workout, be aware of every twist and turn you do. The body responds to your thoughts as well as your movements so focusing on each little squeeze and stretch can make a huge difference. Be constantly aware of the core muscles by drawing the belly button in towards the spine. Not only will this protect against injury but you'll be working those abs with each breathe.

As we are working for 7 minutes we are focusing on quick movements so I have designed the plan to work with body weight only. It is so important to be aware of your form and technique and weights will require a little bit more control. Push hard with every workout without pacing. We want to reach fatigue as quickly as possible. Having said that be vigilant with your posture and once it becomes too difficult to perform the exercise properly move on to the next one. Don't ever substitute a good quality exercise for more reps as this is a sure fire way to injure yourself and create imbalances between the muscle.

How to Use the 7 Minute Workout

Who's it for?

This plan is for anyone who struggles to fit exercise into their daily schedules. Whether you work long hours or have young children the 7 Minute Workout is designed to provide *effective* exercises that can really make a difference. It's all too easy to make excuses about time but for just 7 minutes a day you could improve your health and your body shape drastically.

Who's it not for?

The 7 Minute workout can be done by anyone. Even if you regularly workout the high intensity of these workouts can be a welcome addition to shake up your current plan or simply add a new perspective. If you have fatty trouble zones that you just can't get rid of or you are struggling to increase your running speed then these workouts can help.

Is it better than doing 30 minutes?

If you have time for 30 minutes you are always going to see bigger benefits on a much shorter timescale. I have designed this plan for people who DON'T have time to do 30 minutes a day.

What do I need?

You only need yourself and a stop watch and make sure you always have water on hand.

How should I follow the plan?

There are 3 ways to use this plan:

Follow the book like a diary, working through each day at a time. I recommend this option if you are very new to exercise. If you find week one to be enough of a challenge, keep repeating it until you feel completely read to move on.

If you are quite fit already and have done exercise in the past you may wish to skip week one and start immediately on week two or three.

Simply pick a page and enjoy a different workout every day. You can use the book as a reference for workout ideas for when you have a spare 7 minutes to exercise and you can repeat the workouts as often as you like, so keep it interesting.

Good Luck!

The 7 steps to healthy eating

Fat loss begins in the kitchen and the key to any workout program is healthy nutrition. I come across many clients who work long hours who claim they honestly don't have the energy to exercise after a hard day at the office. The solution is simple; a clean eating plan that focuses on natural foods. Not only will your energy levels improve your skin will look and feel better, you'll feel less fatigued in the afternoons and you will also sleep well.

1) Week 1: Eat as much white meat, fish, vegetables and fruit as you want, except bananas. Aim to eat more vegetables than fruit as fruit contains a lot of sugar.

Have a fist full of nuts and seeds a day. (Milled flax seeds are a good choice)

You can have eggs, herbal tea and coconut water. You may also have corn, sweet potato and other root vegetables but **not** potatoes

No dairy, alcohol, refined carbohydrates (read below), sugar, red meat, caffeine or packaged foods. (It sounds harsh but you'll survive!)

2) Week 2 and 3: As above but you can add in a fistful of carbohydrates on Monday, Wednesday and Friday.

This should follow on from your hardest HIIT workout routines.

Choose from this list ONLY:

Brown Rice

Oats

Quinoa

Cous Cous

3) Eliminate these foods from your life:

Dairy- Just for the first week. You will get all your calcium from green vegetables. If you are concerned about adequate amounts try a supplement as well but this is not compulsory.

 Caffeine- (except green tea) Caffeine increases the effects of cortisol and actually stores fat around your middle. Replace with herbal teas such as Liquorice tea which is great for stabilising a sweet tooth and mint tea which can calm discomfort during digestion.

Refined carbohydrates- White pasta, biscuits, chocolates, bread, noodles, cereal, crackers (or anything that contains wheat)

Processed sugar- Anything with syrup or sweetener and anything ending in 'ose'. Avoid artificial sweeteners.

Ready meals- and pre packaged meals. These are very high in salt and empty calories. Everything should be fresh and natural.

4) Drink plenty of water.

All chemical reactions in the body take place in water including calorie burning. Dehydration causes the body to fatigue and reduces the capacity for fat reduction; it will also decrease concentration, efficiency and increases the effects of ageing.

Drink a pint of cold water every morning and half an hour before lunch and dinner and aim for at least 6 glasses a day. Once you feel thirsty you are already dehydrated. Place a reminder on your phone to go off at regular intervals to remind you to grab a drink and keep a bottle of water in your bag or at your desk.

5) Include at every meal:

Protein- Portion size about a hands span worth

Lean chicken, turkey, duck, quorn,

Free range eggs

Fish-Tuna, smoked mackerel, kippers, salmon, prawns, mussels, squid, halibut (pretty much any white fish)

Raw nuts-Walnuts, Brazils, almonds, macadamia nuts, pecans, flax seeds, sesame seeds, pumpkin and sunflower seeds.

Beans and lentils

Raw nut butters

Fat sources-

Extra virgin olive oil

Fish oil

Cod liver oil (supplement or liquid)

Flax seeds

Avocadoes

Coconut oil

Raw nuts

Fibrous carbohydrates: Portion 2/3 of your plate should be green vegetables

All vegetables

All fruits

6) Eat little and often

Including a mid morning and mid afternoon snack. This will ensure your metabolism keeps ticking over and avoids that 4pm slump.

Try one of these options:

Oat cakes and cottage cheese

A piece of fruit

Vegetable crudités and hummus

A handful of nuts or seeds

Fruit Smoothie

Tbsp of natural yogurt with berries and Agave nectar

7) Don't count calories.

This is a favourite of mine when taking on new clients who have been steadily following 1000 calories a day plan and not losing any weight. Calories are subjective and your body will respond in different ways depending on where the calories are coming from. A 600 calorie meal consisting of vegetables and proteins will be broken down slowly and converted into glycogen for use as energy leaving you fuller for longer. A 600 calorie meal; obtained through a slice of pizza or a chocolate cake will be broken down quickly and contains empty calories that the body cannot convert or use but will instead instantly be stored as fat leaving you hungry and with slightly fuller fat cells. When following an exercise plan such as The 7 Minute Workout you may need more calories to keep the fires burning in order to lose more fat

Ready to go Shopping List

Choose foods from each section. You need to have protein and vegetables at each meal. Complex carbohydrates are only for post workout meals.

Fruit

Apples, Blueberries, Plums, strawberries, Cherries, Mango, Clementine's, watermelon, lemon, pears, bananas, raspberries, melon

Vegetables

Tomatoes, red onion, cucumber, peas, bamboo shoots, kidney beans, broccoli, cauliflower, garlic, avocadoes, peppers, celery, tomatoes, sweet corn, broad beans, green beans, cabbage, celeriac, asparagus, courgettes, mushrooms, squash, leeks, spinach, carrots, onions, chicory, rocket

Dressings

Olive oil, balsamic vinegar, chilli oil, hummus, agave nectar, apple cider vinegar, lemon juice

Complex carbohydrates (post workout)

Cous cous, quinoa, brown rice

Complex carbohydrates (allowed)

Oatcakes

Fresh fish/meat/soya

Tuna, Prawns, salmon, any white fish, lean chicken, lean turkey, tofu, Quorn

Dairy

Eggs, Natural Yogurt

Teas

Green tea, camomile, liquorice, mint, sage, nettle, Echinacea, Tulsi

7 Ways to stay healthy when eating out

In the corporate world it is very common to eat out on a regular basis and I also have clients who simply cannot be bothered to cook after a long day at the office and will eat take out at least two or three times a week. It is important to make healthy choices when eating out this often as rich foods combined with big restaurant portions can play havoc with your waistline.

Restaurants

1) If drinking wine, have a glass of water between each glass to fill you up.

2) Try to avoid eating the bread rolls whilst waiting for your dinner to be served, ask for a small side salad instead.

3) Once your meal is served eat a portion of protein which is approximately the size of your hand with double the amount in vegetables and if you want to have a dessert, then don't eat any complex carbohydrates with your main course.

Takeaway

At Chinese restaurants avoid deep fried items such as spring rolls/ fried noodles/ crispy meats and sweet and sour items and try boiled rather than fried rice.

At Indian restaurants avoid Kormas, creamy sauces or anything fried or dipped in butter. Tikka, Tandoori, Pilau rice and Naan bread without butter are better choices.

Fast Food

6) Burgers tend to be lower in fat than chicken fish sandwiches, but order burgers without mayonnaise or sauce and avoid extra cheese as this significantly increases the fat content.

7) Go for salad instead of chips as a side option.

7 Day Menu Plan

Day 1

Breakfast- Plain natural yogurt and fresh berries (if you need a sweet kick add some agave nectar)

Lunch- Mixed green salad with tuna and quinoa (This can be cooked veg as well!)

Dinner- Roasted vegetables (broccoli/carrots/garlic/peppers/cauliflower/courgettes/baby sweet corn) with lean piece of chicken and mashed butterbeans.

Day 2

Breakfast- Boiled egg with rye bread and a piece of fresh fruit.

Lunch- Mixed bean and veg soup (Covent Garden soup/Tesco veg soup) Piece of fruit.

Dinner- Brown rice with chicken, onions and garlic fried with peppers, green beans and tomatoes

Day 3

Breakfast – Fresh berries with natural yogurt (agave nectar if necessary)

Lunch- Beetroot and green leaves with sunflower and pumpkin seeds and handful of prawns. Fruit smoothie for afters (Handful of Raspberries, 1 apple, 1 banana, 1 orange and as much spinach and kale as you can squeeze in. Add apple juice for consistency)

Dinner- Fillet of fish (unbattered!) with spinach and asparagus sprinkled with lemon and cupful of brown rice.

Day 4

Breakfast- rye bread with marmite, boiled egg and piece of fruit.

Lunch- Green salad with chicken strips, avocado and Clementine pieces. Fruit smoothie as above.

 Dinner- Mushroom stir fry (beansprouts/carrots/onions/garlic/chillis/asparagus/mushrooms/green beans/mange tout/baby sweet corn) with king prawns and butterbean mash.

Day 5

Breakfast- Cottage cheese on oat cakes with piece of fresh fruit and handful of walnuts.

Lunch- Green soup and oat cakes (In a pan fry 1 onion, 1 stick of celery and garlic with extra virgin olive oil till brown. Add 1 litre of veg stock, 1 courgette, 1 bunch of broccoli, 250g of asparagus, 250g of green beans, and 180g of spinach and bring to boil. Blend to create smooth soup) takes 15 minutes.

Dinner- Oven cooked salmon with steamed veg (broccoli/asparagus/spinach/carrots).

Day 6

Breakfast-Berry compote (blueberries/ raspberries/ strawberries and red berries with natural plain yogurt)

Lunch- Balsamic chicken salad (Green beans/roasted peppers/tomatoes/boneless, skinless chicken breast and balsamic vinegar)

Dinner- Tomatoes minestrone soup Carrot, celery and apple salad with sliced grilled chicken and natural yogurt.

Day 7

Cheat day! Having a cheat day once a week will stop you feeling so deprived and allow you to treat yourself within reason. Treat yourself to a slice of cake or a couple of pieces of pizza but don't go overboard.

The sudden shock of extra glucose in the body will help to regenerate the metabolism and stop the body reaching a plateau. This is due to the release of hormones. Leptin is a hormone which controls many metabolic processes in your body and it is also responsible for fat loss. The more leptin you have the faster you lose fat. The silly thing is the more fat you lose the lower your leptin levels which is why it is so hard to lose the last few lbs.

Leptin is produced in fat cells so the smaller you are and the fewer fat cells, the less leptin you'll produce.

When you restrict calories you reduce leptin. Despite what you may think we are not trying to restrict calories on this plan, however I am not asking you to reduce calories I am just encouraging you to get them from cleaner, higher energy foods.

Whilst doing this if we constantly regulate our leptin levels fat loss will be quicker. This is where cheat days come in. When you eat the foods that are high in extra calories that you're body doesn't need you will increase the amount of leptin produced in fat cells and kick start that fat burning furnace for another week!

7 Minutes to combat Stress

Exercise has been proven to have a positive impact on stress relief and just 7 minutes a day can drastically improve your mood. Stress is a natural response to a stimulus i.e. an important deadline or an exam. The body enters a fight or flight response phase which in the short term can help us push through the difficulties, forcing us to meet those deadlines or making sure we study for the exam. However repeated exposure to high levels of stress can have a negative impact on our health by raising the blood pressure, increasing the risk of cardiovascular disease and even speeding up the ageing process.

We have previously spoken about cortisol, this is a stress hormone secreted by the adrenal gland to help raise blood sugar levels when the body is in crisis. Cortisol does have a few positive effects including regulating the metabolism, improving memory function and increasing immunity. However when the body reaches a state of chronic stress, cortisol levels in the blood stream can reach high levels for a prolonged period of time. High levels of cortisol have been shown to inhibit fat loss, slow down thyroid function, slow down cognitive processes and break down lean muscle mass.

To maintain a healthy lifestyle it is important to keep stress levels under control. To do this its important to be aware when the body enters a fight or flight response phase. Symptoms may include shortness of breath, headaches, impaired vision, and stomach pains or in the long term difficulty sleeping, weight gain and high cholesterol.

Once you have entered the fight or flight phase we need to switch the body to relaxation mode and this could simply be taking some deep breaths, closing your eyes and counting to 10 or sitting down to a hot cup of tea to simply regroup.

Stress is a form of repressed energy that has nowhere to go, so instead stress hormones such as cortisol are released to convert this energy to elsewhere in the body. Exercise enables this energy to be released as heat and water so even just 7 Minutes of high intensity exercise can lower cortisol levels and instead create lean muscle mass. The more muscle mass we have the more energy we use at rest helping us to cope with stressful situations.

 Going back to being 'aware' as we exercise, it is important to focus on each movement to create a mind, body balance switching off the outside world and inciting an 'inner calm'.

Pilates and Yoga can also have the same effect. Connecting your movement to your mind and taking the time to breathe deeply floods the body with oxygen, lowers the heart rate and blood pressure and massages the internal organs.

If you need a slightly calmer routine to stretch out the muscles and calm the mind try this 7 Minute Pilates and stretch routine. Try it before bed to help you sleep or first thing in the morning to release any tension before work.

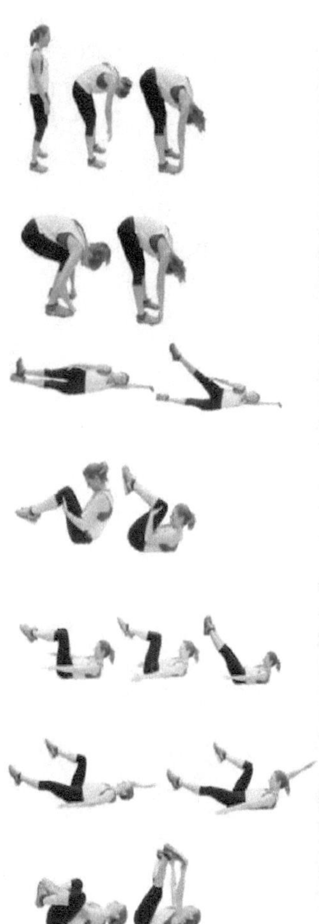

1) Roll down- Stand tall and inhale. Exhale and tuck chin to chest, slowly rolling one vertebrae at a time towards the floor. Let arms hang loose and keeps knees soft. Once you reach the floor inhale and exhale to re-stack the spine one vertebrae at a time back to ceiling. Repeat X 3

2) Roll down as above then place hands under toes. You may need to bend your knees to do this but keep heels on the floor. Inhale and squat low then exhale to straighten legs as far as you can without letting go of toes and keep looking back through legs. Repeat X 6

3) Side leg lifts- Lay on to one side with bottom arm stretched under the side of the head and relax your neck. Lift both legs off floor keeping hips stacked. Hold and lift the top leg up and down pointing toes up and pushing heel down. X 20 each side

4) Rolling like a Ball- Push to sitting and place hands behind the thighs. Tuck in chin and rock back on to seat bones lifting feet to balance. Inhale and exhale to roll back counting each vertebrae as you go. Immediately roll back to balance. Don't throw neck backwards.
Repeat X 6

5) One Hundred- Lay to floor and lift knees one at a time into table top with knees in line with hips. Imagine your core as a solid square and lift head and shoulders to look through knees. Pulse arms up and down at your sides. If comfortable, extend both legs away. Inhale for 10 pulses then exhale for 10 pulses until you reach 100 beats.

6) Double leg stretch- Keeping knees in table top and head on the floor inhale then extend one leg towards ceiling, reaching opposite arm over the head. If comfortable lift head neck and shoulders to look through knees.
X 20

7) Happy Baby- Reach between knees to grab toes with head resting to the floor. Inhale then exhale to extend legs to ceiling. Repeat X 5

7 Tension Release Exercises you can do in the office

It may not be possible to get down on the office floor and perform a Pilates routine in the middle of the working day so if you do experience high tension levels and need a little release try a few of these little stress relievers!

1) Wrist circles: Stretch the arms out and circle the wrists 10 x in one direction then 10 x in the other.

2) Shoulder lifts: Sit or stand tall and lift the shoulders straight up towards the ears and then let them slide straight back down being aware as you squeeze down the spine (do not roll). 5x

3) Neck rolls: Drop chin to chest and inhale. Roll the head across to one shoulder and then the other (do not tilt head backwards) 4x

4) Knee lifts: Standing or sitting tall, lift alternate knees bracing abdominals as you lift. 10x

5) Stand to sit: An alternative to a squat, sit down then continue to stand and sit keeping arms out in front of you and weight in heels 5 x

6) Arm reaches: Whilst sitting reach alternate arms up and over head leaning from side to side 6 x

7) Trunk twists: Sit tall and twist from side to side (as though twisting a lid of a jar) engaging the core.

Plan your workout

To succeed in any business venture it is vital to plan a schedule. Nobody trying to run a business will head to the office without planning the meetings or interviews they need to do that day and writing them in a diary.

Therefore to succeed in any fitness plan it is necessary to plan your workouts and schedule them into your day exactly as if they were an important meeting.

If you're naturally organized this won't feel like too much of a task but for those of you who tend to wing your exercise sessions it's time to get serious. Write your 7 Minute workout into your diary. Schedule it for when you wake up or before you go to bed or place it during your lunch break. Having it scheduled into your day will make it a priority.

If you need extra encouragement place a post it note on your bedside mirror or on the fridge or even on your lunch box (if you have one!) to remind yourself to do your workout.

Create a goals table covering 7 days for 3 weeks. A sample is provided below. Write down a goal for the end of each week, for example; 'Lose 2lbs this week' or 'increase my reps by 3 for each exercise'.

Each day, tick off if you have done your workout and also state if you had any slip ups with food. It might sound tedious but it takes 10 seconds and will really help to keep you on track and motivated.

	Mon	Tues	Weds	Thurs	Fri	Sat	Sun
Week 1							
Week 2							
Week 3							

7 Days to Wake up those Muscles

During this first week we will focus on exercise to wake up the largest fat burning muscles including the gluteus and abdominals and concentrate on realigning the body. **How to**: Each workout will consist of 7 exercises done for 1 minute each. If you spend long hours at a desk your muscles may be sleeping and inactive and launching into a full on exercise plan without recruiting the right areas is pointless. Use this week to become really aware of your body, pay attention as we lift and squeeze as muscles respond to your thoughts as well as your movements. Everything should be moving and awake!

This week is vital if you are new to exercise however if you are more experienced you may wish to skip week one and move straight to week 2.

Day 1

"Life is either a daring adventure or nothing" **Helen Keller**

Quick Tip: Keep a pair of trainers and a workout kit in a cupboard or desk drawer at work so you can fit your workout at lunch or straight after work. This will make sure you stick to the plan without giving you time to come up with excuses.

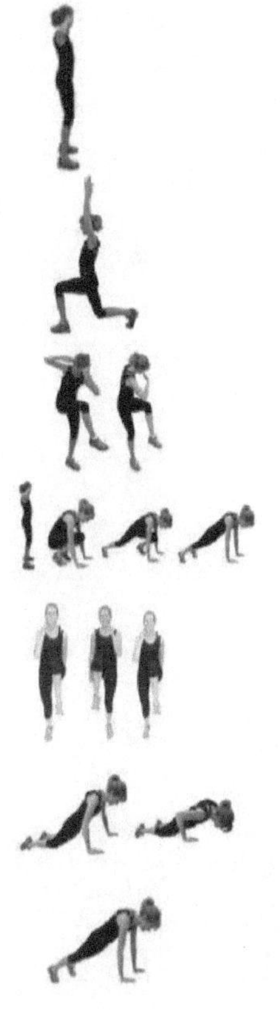

Perform each exercise for 1 minute with no rest in between

1) Glute Squeezes- Stand tall with hands to head. Tense bottom muscles and squeeze shoulder blades together. Hold for 10's then relax for 10's. Repeat for 1 minutes

2) Lunges- Lift arms up to the ceiling so arms are level with your ears. Step alternate feet forwards bending back knee. Make each move explosive and fast.

4) Criss Cross- Place hands to head and quickly rotate opposite elbow to knee pulling in the belly button.

3) Inch Worm Burpee- Place hands to floor and step one leg at a time back into plank position. Step back towards hands one at a time and come up to standing squeezing shoulders back.

5) 1-2-3- Stand tall and quickly lift knees high jogging from side to side in the beat of 1-2-3, 1-2-3

6) Kneeling press up- Place hands wide and keep knees on the floor. Leading with the nose lower the torso towards the floor and forcefully push up.

7) Extended plank hold- Place hands under shoulders and extend the legs out. Push forwards on the toes and hold.

Glute Squeezes

Lunges

Criss Cross

Inch Worm Burpee

1-2-3

Kneeling Press Up

Plank

Day 2

'The Surest Way not to fail is to determine to succeed' **Richard Brinsley Sheridan**

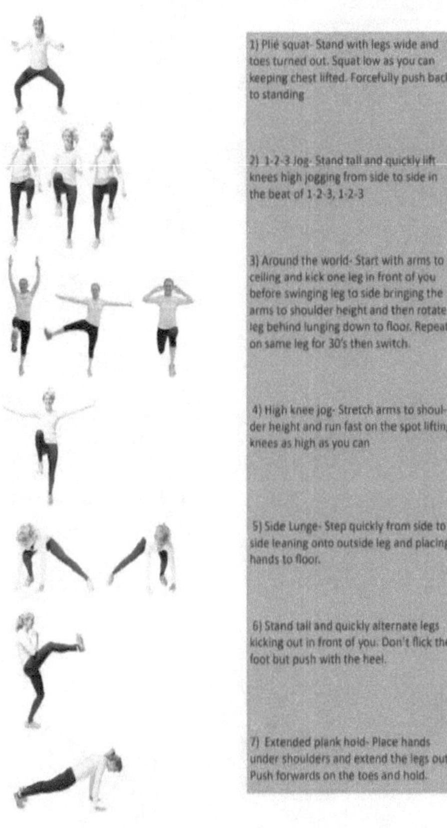

1) Plié squat- Stand with legs wide and toes turned out. Squat low as you can keeping chest lifted. Forcefully push back to standing

2) 1-2-3 Jog- Stand tall and quickly lift knees high jogging from side to side in the beat of 1-2-3, 1-2-3

3) Around the world- Start with arms to ceiling and kick one leg in front of you before swinging leg to side bringing the arms to shoulder height and then rotate leg behind lunging down to floor. Repeat on same leg for 30's then switch.

4) High knee jog- Stretch arms to shoulder height and run fast on the spot lifting knees as high as you can

5) Side Lunge- Step quickly from side to side leaning onto outside leg and placing hands to floor.

6) Stand tall and quickly alternate legs kicking out in front of you. Don't flick the foot but push with the heel.

7) Extended plank hold- Place hands under shoulders and extend the legs out. Push forwards on the toes and hold.

Plié Squat

1-2-3

Around the World

High Knees

Side Lunge

Flick Kicks

Plank

Day 3

<u>Quick Tip:</u> Don't feel guilty for cheating. Designate one day a week to treat yourself to that slice of cake or the pizza you have been craving. Leptin is a hormone responsible for fat loss and is secreted by the fat cells. As we lose weight leptin levels reduce so if we cheat on the healthy eating every once in a while we can kick start the leptin levels and initiate faster fat burn!

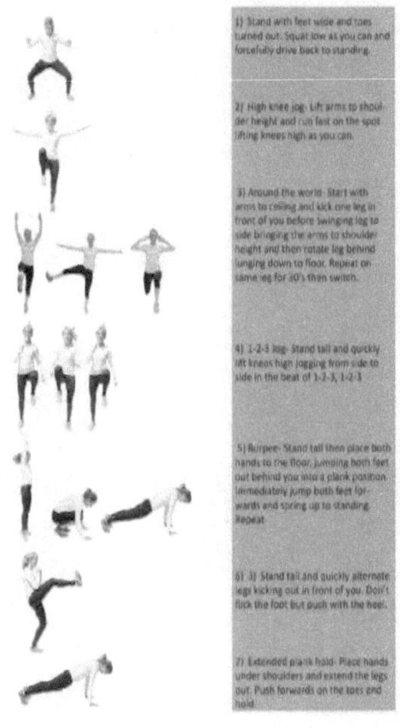

1) Stand with feet wide and toes turned out. Squat low as you can and forcefully drive back to standing.

2) High knee jog- Lift arms to shoulder height and run fast on the spot lifting knees high as you can.

3) Around the world- Start with arms to ceiling and kick one leg in front of you before swinging leg to side bringing the arms to shoulder height and then rotate leg behind lunging down to floor. Repeat on same leg for 30's then switch.

4) 1-2-3 Jog- Stand tall and quickly lift knees high jogging from side to side in the beat of 1-2-3, 1-2-3

5) Burpee- Stand tall then place both hands to the floor, jumping both feet out behind you into a plank position. Immediately jump both feet forwards and spring up to standing. Repeat

6) 3) Stand tall and quickly alternate legs kicking out in front of you. Don't flick the foot but push with the heel.

7) Extended plank hold- Place hands under shoulders and extend the legs out. Push forwards on the toes and hold.

Plié Squat
High Knees
Around the World
1-2-3
Burpee
Flick Kicks
Plank

Day 4

"If you have an hour, will you not improve that hour, instead of idling it away?" **Lord Chesterfield**

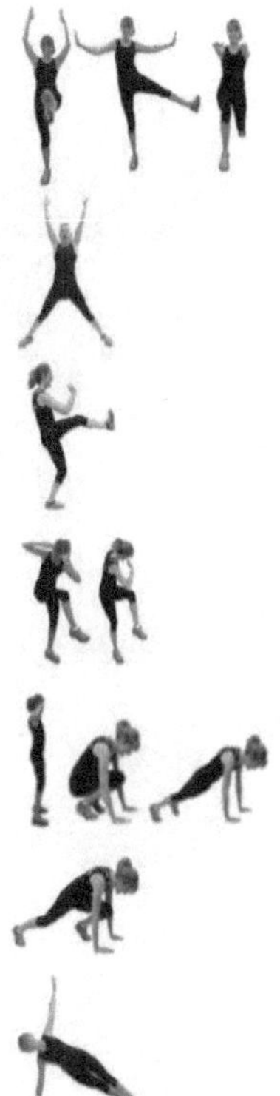

1) 1)Start with arms in front you and kick one leg in front before swinging leg to side and bringing arms to shoulders and then rotate the leg behind lunging down to floor. Repeat on one leg for 30's then switch.

2) Star Jump- Stand tall and quickly jump arms and legs wide coming off the floor.

3) Stand tall and quickly alternate legs kicking out in front of you. Don't flick the foot but push with the heel.

4) Criss Cross- Place hands to head and quickly rotate opposite elbow to knee pulling in the belly button.

5) Burpee- Stand tall then place both hands to the floor, jumping both feet out behind you into a plank position. Immediately jump both feet forwards and spring up to standing. Repeat

6) Mountain Climbers- Place hands under shoulders and stretch into a plank position pushing bodyweight forwards. Run legs in and out quickly.

7) Side plank- Sit on to side with weight on one arm and top leg place in front of the bottom leg. Lift hips reaching the arm to the ceiling. Gently lower to the floor and repeat.

Around the World
Star Jumps
Flick Kicks
Criss Cross
Burpee
Mountain Climbers
Side Plank

Day 5

"Look back at a day when you were supremely satisfied at the end. It's not a day when you lounged around doing nothing, it was when you had everything to do and you've done it." **Margaret Thatcher**

Quick Tip: When in the office stand up whilst on the phone and move around. If you're in your own office or booth do some squats or lunges whilst on the phone (nobody can see you!)

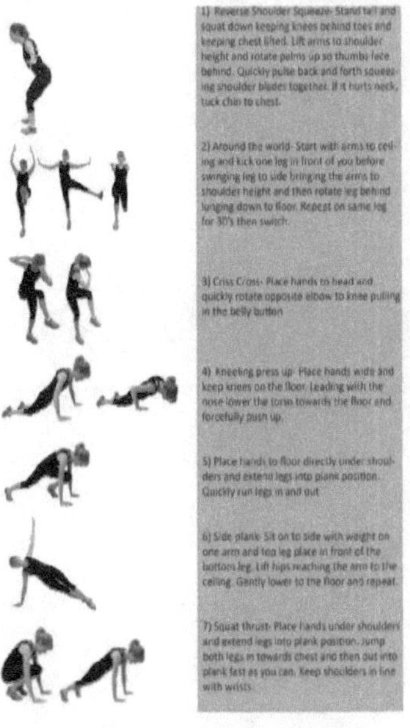

1) Reverse Shoulder Squeeze- Stand tall and squat down keeping knees behind toes and keeping chest lifted. Lift arms to shoulder height and rotate palms up so thumbs face behind. Quickly pulse back and forth squeezing shoulder blades together. If it hurts neck, tuck chin to chest.

2) Around the world- Start with arms to ceiling and kick one leg in front of you before swinging leg to side bringing the arms to shoulder height and then rotate leg behind lunging down to floor. Repeat on same leg for 30's then switch.

3) Criss Cross- Place hands to head and quickly rotate opposite elbow to knee pulling in the belly button

4) Kneeling press up- Place hands wide and keep knees on the floor. Leading with the nose lower the torso towards the floor and forcefully push up.

5) Place hands to floor directly under shoulders and extend legs into plank position. Quickly run legs in and out

6) Side plank- Sit on to side with weight on one arm and top leg place in front of the bottom leg. Lift hips reaching the arm to the ceiling. Gently lower to the floor and repeat.

7) Squat thrust- Place hands under shoulders and extend legs into plank position. Jump both legs in towards chest and then out into plank fast as you can. Keep shoulders in line with wrists.

<u>Reverse Shoulder Squeeze</u>

<u>Around the World</u>

<u>Criss Cross</u>

<u>Kneeling Press Up</u>

<u>Mountain Climbers</u>

<u>Side Plank</u>

<u>Squat Thrust</u>

Day 6

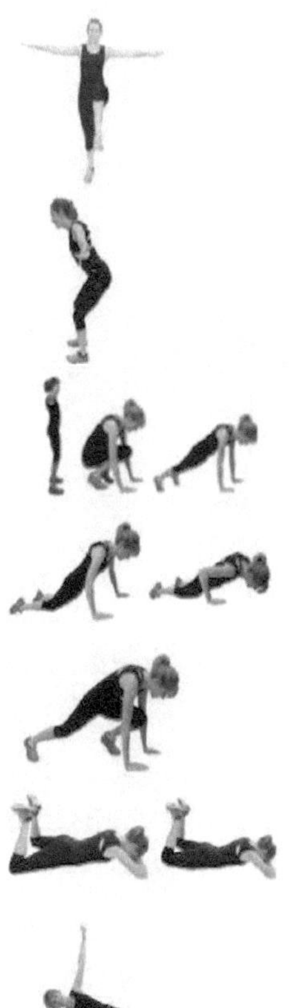

1) High knee jog- Lift arms to shoulder height and run fast on the spot lifting knees high as you can.

2) Reverse Shoulder Squeeze- Stand tall and squat down keeping knees behind toes and keeping chest lifted. Lift arms to shoulder height and rotate palms up so thumbs face behind. Quickly pulse back and forth squeezing shoulder blades together. If it hurts neck, tuck chin to chest.

3) Burpee- Stand tall then place both hands to the floor, jumping both feet out behind you into a plank position. Immediately jump both feet forwards and spring up to standing. Repeat

4) Kneeling press up- Place hands wide and keep knees on the floor. Leading with the nose lower the torso towards the floor and forcefully push up.

5) Place hands to floor directly under shoulders and extend legs into plank position. Quickly run legs in and out

6) Lying glute squeezes- Lay on front with hands under forehead and knees bent. Take knees wide but press heels together. Pressing heels as hard as you can and squeezing bottom muscles push feet towards ceiling lifting knees then gently lower. Keep shoulders relaxed throughout.

7) Side plank- Sit on to side with weight on one arm and top leg place in front of the bottom leg. Lift hips reaching the arm to the ceiling. Gently lower to the floor and repeat.

"The key to change… is to let go of fear." **Rosanne Cash**

<u>High Knees</u>
<u>Reverse Shoulder Squeeze</u>
<u>Burpee</u>
<u>Kneeling Press Up</u>
<u>Mountain Climbers</u>
<u>Lying Glute Squeezes</u>
<u>Side Plank</u>

Day 7

The surest way not to fail is to determine to succeed. **Richard Brinsley Sheridan**

Quick Tip: Try Body brushing every night before bed or before a shower helps to boost the circulation. Brush toward the heart to by to eliminate wastes and toxins, the source of stubborn cellulite. Skin brushing may reduce fat deposits, tightening skin and toning muscles. It sloughs off dead skin cells, leaving your skin soft and smooth. According to Yoga Journal, skin brushing may stimulate the lymphatic system, which boosts immunity.

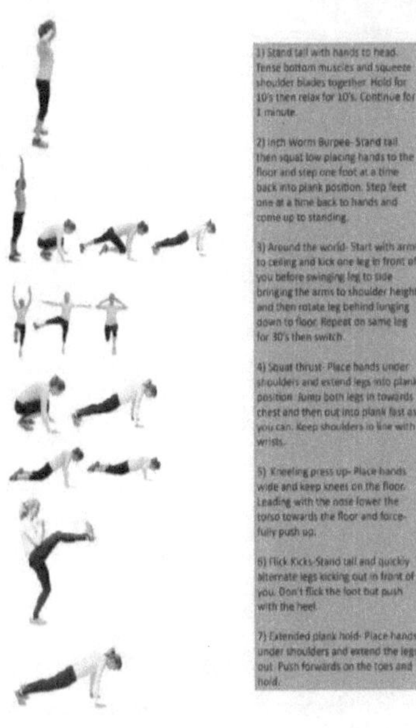

Glute Squeezes

Inch Worm Burpee

Around the World
Squat Thrust
Kneeling Press Up
Flick Kicks
Plank

7 Days to Ramp up the Intensity

Over the next 7 days we will continue to build on the muscles we have re awoken and will start to burn, tone and define. This week relies on high impact exercises so continue to use your awareness and feel each muscle as we use it. Aim to push harder and watch the sweat drip off you after each routine. If you don't feel ready for this yet return to the start of week one and repeat.

How to: Each routine follows the same pattern. Repeat the first 4 exercises as a circuit doing 20's flat out on each with 10's rest in between. Do the circuit 3 x non-stop. The finisher is 1 minute flat out.

Day 8

"Without discipline there is no life at all" **Katherine Hepburn**

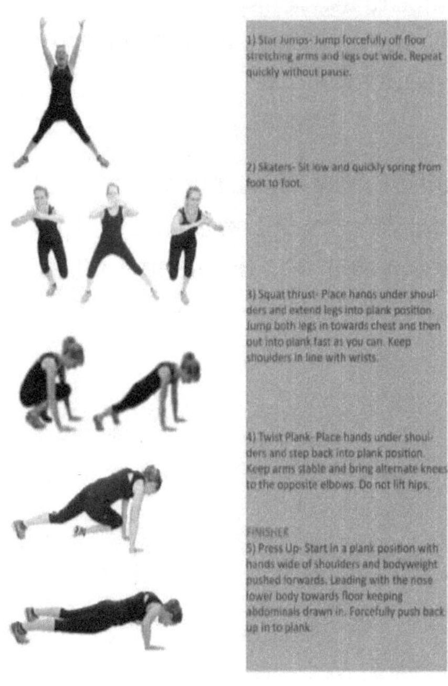

1) Star Jumps- Jump forcefully off floor stretching arms and legs out wide. Repeat quickly without pause.

2) Skaters- Sit low and quickly spring from foot to foot.

3) Squat thrust- Place hands under shoulders and extend legs into plank position. Jump both legs in towards chest and then out into plank fast as you can. Keep shoulders in line with wrists.

4) Twist Plank- Place hands under shoulders and step back into plank position. Keep arms stable and bring alternate knees to the opposite elbows. Do not lift hips.

FINISHER
5) Press Up- Start in a plank position with hands wide of shoulders and bodyweight pushed forwards. Leading with the nose lower body towards floor keeping abdominals drawn in. Forcefully push back up in to plank.

<u>Star Jumps</u>
<u>Skaters</u>
<u>Squat Thrust</u>
<u>Twist Plank</u>
<u>Press Ups</u>

Day 9

Quick Tip: Remove all fatty, sugary foods from your house. Avoid cafes or places you may be tempted to have sweets and put some nuts or raisins in your handbag for when you need a snack on the go.

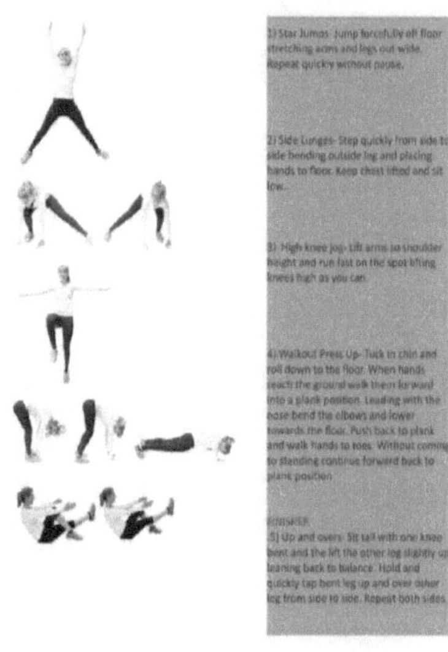

<u>Star Jumps</u>
<u>Side lunge</u>
<u>High Knees</u>
<u>Walkout Press Up</u>
<u>Up and Over's</u>

Day 10

"Thoughts are but dreams, till their effects be tried"

William Shakespeare

Quick Tip: When having your post workout shower turn the tap to cold for the last 30's and let it pound on the back of your neck. We have 2 types of fat brown and white. Brown fat activity increases with cold temperature exposure. Brown fat uses calories from normal fat, or white fat, and burns it for fuel. An increase in brown fat

activity may allow a person to burn an extra 500 calories per day.

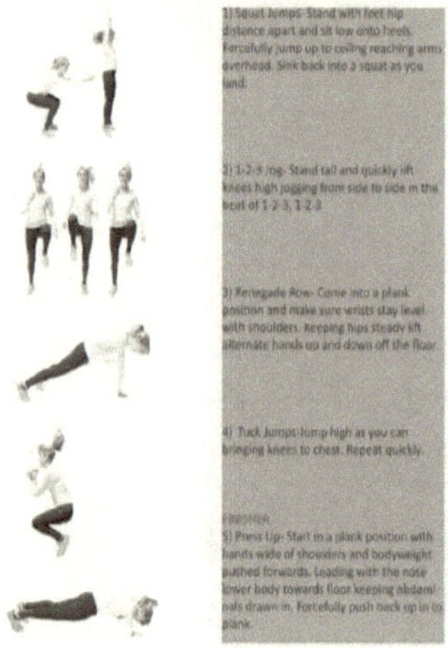

<u>Squat Jumps</u>
<u>1-2-3</u>
<u>Renegade Row</u>
<u>Tuck Jumps</u>
<u>Press Ups</u>

Day 11

I hated every minute of training, but I said, 'Don't quit. Suffer now and live the rest of your life as a champion.' **Muhammad Ali**

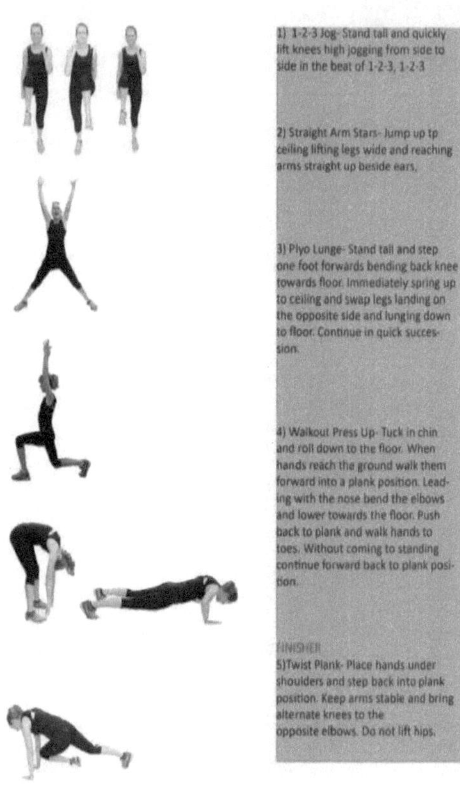

1) 1-2-3 Jog- Stand tall and quickly lift knees high jogging from side to side in the beat of 1-2-3, 1-2-3

2) Straight Arm Stars- Jump up tp ceiling lifting legs wide and reaching arms straight up beside ears,

3) Plyo Lunge- Stand tall and step one foot forwards bending back knee towards floor. Immediately spring up to ceiling and swap legs landing on the opposite side and lunging down to floor. Continue in quick succession.

4) Walkout Press Up- Tuck in chin and roll down to the floor. When hands reach the ground walk them forward into a plank position. Leading with the nose bend the elbows and lower towards the floor. Push back to plank and walk hands to toes. Without coming to standing continue forward back to plank position.

FINISHER
5)Twist Plank- Place hands under shoulders and step back into plank position. Keep arms stable and bring alternate knees to the opposite elbows. Do not lift hips.

<u>1-2-3</u>
<u>Straight Arm Stars</u>
<u>Lunges</u>
<u>Walkout Press Up</u>
<u>Twist Plank</u>

Day 12

"If you don't like something, change it. If you can't change it, change your attitude. Don't complain." **Maya Angelou**

Quick Tip: Put an uplifting playlist on your iPod. Any music with a beat over 130bpm will speed up your workout and push you to work harder. Listen to music on your walk to work, you'll probably find you get there 5 minutes earlier!

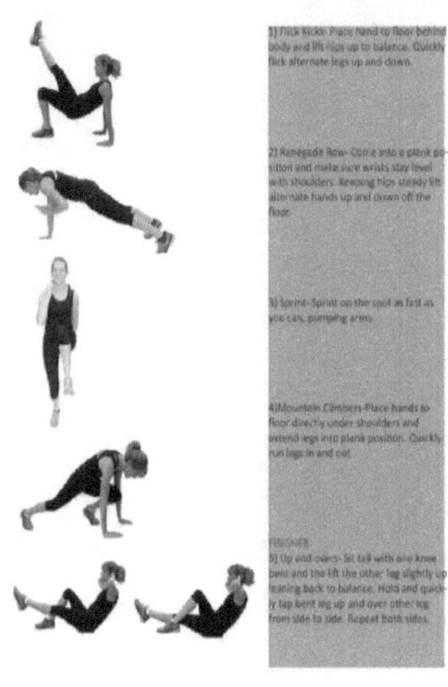

<u>Sitting Flick Kicks</u>
<u>Renegade Row</u>
<u>Sprint</u>
<u>Mountain Climbers</u>
<u>Up and Over's</u>

Day 13

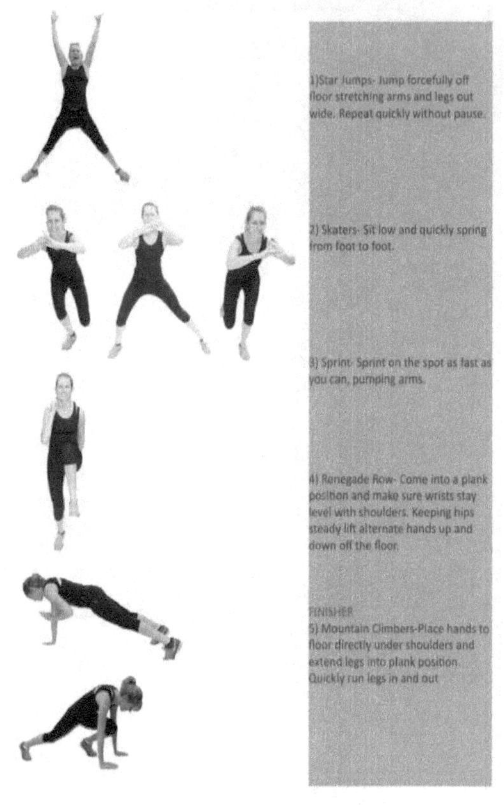

1)Star Jumps- Jump forcefully off floor stretching arms and legs out wide. Repeat quickly without pause.

2) Skaters- Sit low and quickly spring from foot to foot.

3) Sprint- Sprint on the spot as fast as you can, pumping arms.

4) Renegade Row- Come into a plank position and make sure wrists stay level with shoulders. Keeping hips steady lift alternate hands up and down off the floor.

FINISHER
5) Mountain Climbers-Place hands to floor directly under shoulders and extend legs into plank position. Quickly run legs in and out

<u>Star Jumps</u>
<u>Skaters</u>
<u>Sprint</u>
<u>Renegade Row</u>
<u>Mountain Climbers</u>

Day 14

Quick Tip: For a quick simple breakfast mix 2 eggs with a banana and create banana pancakes. Serve with blueberries and raspberries for an antioxidant energy boost.

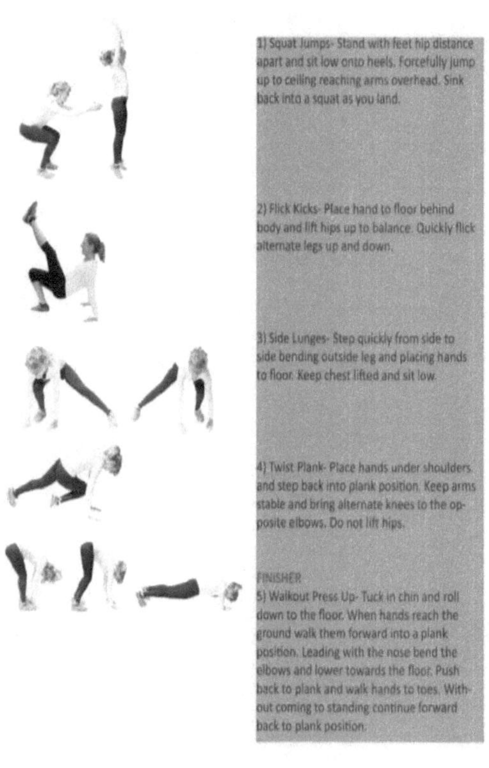

Squat Jumps

Flick Kicks

Side lunge

Twist plank

Walkout Press Up

7 Days to feel the burn

This is our hardest week yet with all the routines featuring short sharp twists and turns and lots of impact. Make every move punchy and forceful and once more be aware of every muscle. Consciously squeeze and tense to make sure each muscle is awake. The exercises in this round are a little more advanced so only continue if you feel ready. If not return to week two.

How To: Each Routine consists of 3 pairs of exercises with a 1 Minute finisher.

Start with Pair A, doing both exercises back to back for 30's each then take a 10's break. Repeat Pair A then move to Pair B, then pair C and so on. Do the finisher for 1 minute flat out.

Day 15

Quick Tip: Plan your food shopping trips. Make a list and DO NOT deviate. This will save time and stop you from filling the basket with unwanted sugary treats. Eat before you go so you are not tempted to snack while you shop.

If you have the means try a healthy home delivery service such as Graze.com or Bodychef.com

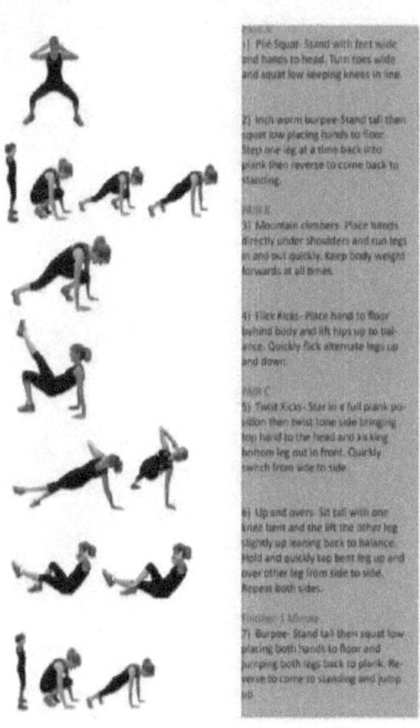

PHASE A

1) Plié Squat- Stand with feet wide and hands to head. Turn toes wide and squat low keeping knees in line.

2) Inch worm burpee-Stand tall then squat low placing hands to floor. Step one leg at a time back into plank then reverse to come back to standing.

PHASE B

3) Mountain climbers- Place hands directly under shoulders and run legs in and out quickly. Keep body weight forwards at all times.

4) Flick Kicks- Place hand to floor behind body and lift hips up to balance. Quickly flick alternate legs up and down.

PHASE C

5) Twist Kicks- Start in a full plank position then twist to one side bringing top hand to the head and kicking bottom leg out in front. Quickly switch from side to side.

6) Up and overs- Sit tall with one knee bent and the lift the other leg slightly up leaning back to balance. Hold and quickly tap bent leg up and over other leg from side to side. Repeat both sides.

Finisher 1 Minute

7) Burpee- Stand tall then squat low placing both hands to floor and jumping both legs back to plank. Reverse to come to standing and jump up

<u>Plié Squat</u>
<u>Inch Worm Burpee</u>
<u>Mountain Climbers</u>
<u>Flick Kicks</u>
<u>Twist and Kick</u>
<u>Up and Over's</u>
<u>Burpee</u>

Day 16

"If you don't do what's best for your body, you're the one who comes up on the short end". **Julius Erving**

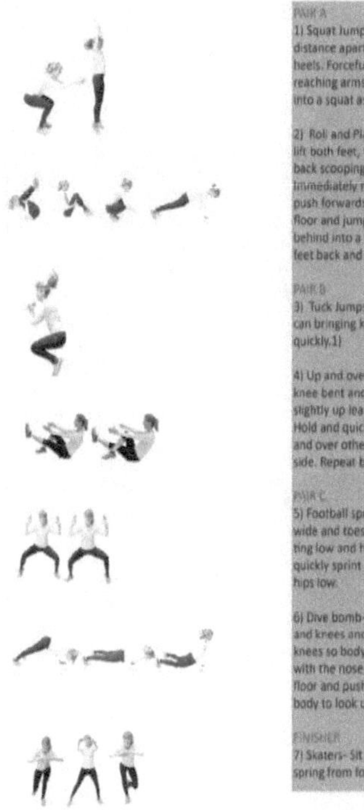

PAIR A

1) Squat Jumps- Stand with feet hip distance apart and sit low onto heels. Forcefully jump up to ceiling reaching arms overhead. Sink back into a squat as you land.

2) Roll and Plank- Sit on floor and lift both feet, tucking in chin roll back scooping in the belly button. Immediately roll back to sitting and push forwards placing hands to the floor and jumping both legs out behind into a plank position. Jump feet back and reverse the move.

PAIR B

3) Tuck Jumps-Jump high as you can bringing knees to chest. Repeat quickly.1)

4) Up and overs- Sit tall with one knee bent and the lift the other leg slightly up leaning back to balance. Hold and quickly tap bent leg up and over other leg from side to side. Repeat both sides.

PAIR C

5) Football sprint- Stand with feet wide and toes turned out, squatting low and hold. Lift heels and quickly sprint on the spot keeping hips low.

6) Dive bomb- Come onto hands and knees and curling toes lift knees so body forms a v. Leading with the nose lower chest to the floor and push forwards curving body to look up. Reverse.

FINISHER

7) Skaters- Sit low and quickly spring from foot to foot.

Squat Jump

Roll and Plank

Tuck Jump

Up and Overs

Football Sprint

Dive Bomb

Skaters

Day 17

"You must take personal responsibility. You cannot change the circumstances, the seasons, or the wind, but you can change yourself." **Jim Rohn**

Quick Tip: Protein shakes are a great way to recover after your workout. Try sun Warrior Protein to rebuild and repair muscles. They also act as a great breakfast on the run. Alternatively make a smoothie with egg white or egg white powder.

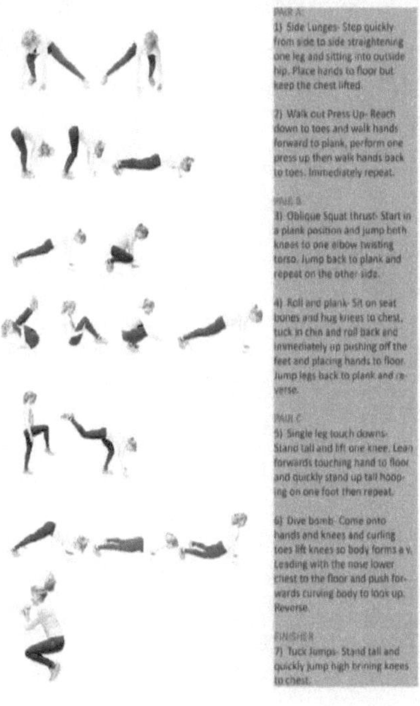

PAIR A:
1) Side Lunges- Step quickly from side to side straightening one leg and sitting into outside hip. Place hands to floor but keep the chest lifted.

2) Walk out Press Up- Reach down to toes and walk hands forward to plank, perform one press up then walk hands back to toes. Immediately repeat.

PAIR B
3) Oblique Squat thrust- Start in a plank position and jump both knees to one elbow twisting torso. Jump back to plank and repeat on the other side.

4) Roll and plank- Sit on seat bones and hug knees to chest, tuck in chin and roll back and immediately up pushing off the feet and placing hands to floor. Jump legs back to plank and re-verse.

PAIR C
5) Single leg touch downs- Stand tall and lift one knee. Lean forwards touching hand to floor and quickly stand up tall hoop-ing on one foot then repeat.

6) Dive bomb- Come onto hands and knees and curling toes lift knees so body forms a v. Leading with the nose lower chest to the floor and push for-wards curving body to look up. Reverse.

FINISHER
7) Tuck Jumps- Stand tall and quickly jump high brining knees to chest.

<u>Side Lunge</u>
<u>Walkout Press Up</u>
<u>Oblique Squat Thrust</u>
<u>Roll and Plank</u>
<u>Single Leg Touch Downs</u>
<u>Dive Bomb</u>
<u>Tuck Jumps</u>

Day 18

"You cannot expect to achieve new goals or move beyond your present circumstances unless you change." **Les Brown**

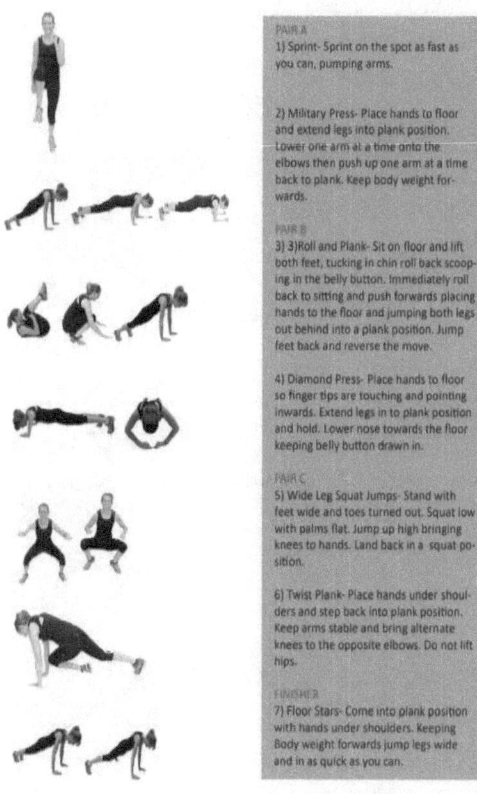

PAIR A

1) Sprint- Sprint on the spot as fast as you can, pumping arms.

2) Military Press- Place hands to floor and extend legs into plank position. Lower one arm at a time onto the elbows then push up one arm at a time back to plank. Keep body weight forwards.

PAIR B

3) 3)Roll and Plank- Sit on floor and lift both feet, tucking in chin roll back scooping in the belly button. Immediately roll back to sitting and push forwards placing hands to the floor and jumping both legs out behind into a plank position. Jump feet back and reverse the move.

4) Diamond Press- Place hands to floor so finger tips are touching and pointing inwards. Extend legs in to plank position and hold. Lower nose towards the floor keeping belly button drawn in.

PAIR C

5) Wide Leg Squat Jumps- Stand with feet wide and toes turned out. Squat low with palms flat. Jump up high bringing knees to hands. Land back in a squat position.

6) Twist Plank- Place hands under shoulders and step back into plank position. Keep arms stable and bring alternate knees to the opposite elbows. Do not lift hips.

FINISHER

7) Floor Stars- Come into plank position with hands under shoulders. Keeping Body weight forwards jump legs wide and in as quick as you can.

<u>Sprint</u>

<u>Military Press</u>

<u>Roll and Plank</u>

<u>Diamond Press</u>

<u>Wide Leg Squat Jump</u>

<u>Twist Plank</u>

<u>Floor Stars</u>

Day 19

"Stand up to your obstacles and do something about them. You will find that they haven't half the strength you think they have." **Norman Vincent Peale**

Quick Tip: Wherever possible, take the stairs! You will activate the glutes, quads, hamstrings, calves and core (all the major muscles that burn lots of calories). Climbing just two flights of stairs everyday could result a loss of 2.7kg or 6lbs per year. Six flights a day could help you trim nearly 18 lbs. Whether it's at work, home, out shopping or a public building take the stairs or walk up the escalator instead of standing still.

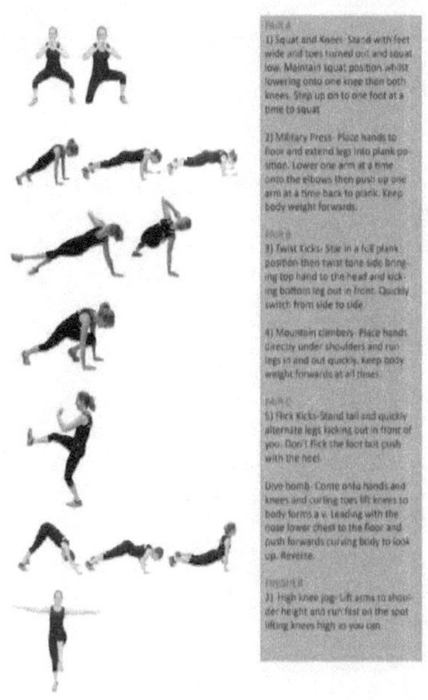

PART A

1) Squat and Kneel- Stand with feet wide and toes turned out and squat low. Maintain squat position whilst lowering onto one knee then both knees. Step up on to one foot at a time to squat

2) Military Press- Place hands to floor and extend legs into plank position. Lower one arm at a time onto the elbows then push up one arm at a time back to plank. Keep body weight forwards.

PART B

3) Twist Kicks- Star in a full plank position then twist tone side bringing top hand to the head and kicking bottom leg out in front. Quickly switch from side to side

4) Mountain climbers- Place hands directly under shoulders and run legs in and out quickly. Keep body weight forwards at all times.

PART C

5) Flick Kicks-Stand tall and quickly alternate legs kicking out in front of you. Don't flick the foot but push with the heel.

Dive-bomb- Come onto hands and knees and curling toes lift knees to body forms a v. Leading with the nose lower chest to the floor and push forwards curving body to look up. Reverse.

FINISHER

3) High knee jog- Lift arms to shoulder height and run fast on the spot lifting knees high as you can

<u>Squat and Kneel</u>

<u>Military Press</u>

<u>Twist and Kick</u>

<u>Mountain Climbers</u>

<u>Flick Kicks</u>

<u>Dive Bomb</u>

<u>High Knee Jog</u>

Day 20

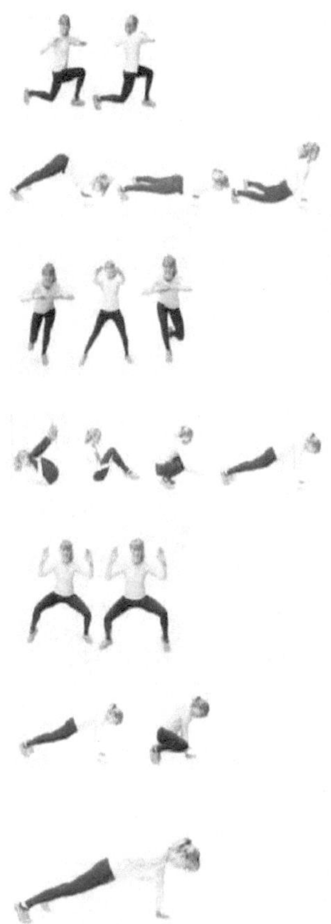

PAIR A

1) Lunge and Twist- Place hands to head and keeping elbows wide step one foot forwards lowering the back knee and twist to look to one side. Forcefully step back to the centre and repeat on the other side.

2) Dive bomb- Come onto hands and knees and curling toes lift knees so body forms a v. Leading with the nose lower chest to the floor and push forwards curving body to look up. Reverse.

PAIR B

3) Skaters- Sit low and quickly spring from foot to foot.

4) Roll and Plank- Sit on floor and lift both feet, tucking in chin roll back scooping in the belly button. Immediately roll back to sitting and push forwards placing hands to the floor and jumping both legs out behind into a plank position. Jump feet back and reverse the move.

PAIR C

5) Football sprint- Stand with feet wide and toes turned out, squatting low and hold. Lift heels and quickly sprint on the spot keeping hips low.

6) Oblique squat thrust- Place hands to floor under shoulders and extend legs into plank position. Quickly jump both legs to one shoulder twisting hips then jump back to centre. Alternate sides.

FINISHER

7) Renegade Row- Come into a plank position and make sure wrists stay level with shoulders. Keeping hips steady lift alternate hands up and down off the floor.

Great things are not done by impulse, but by a series of small things brought together."
Vincent Van Gogh

Lunge and Twist
Dive Bomb
Skaters
Roll and Plank
Football Sprint
Oblique Squat Thrust
Renegade Row

Day 21

"The time for action is now. It's never too late to do something" **Carl Sandburg.**

Quick Tip: If you feel guilty for taking time out to exercise when you should be working, try downloading work onto an iPad or phone so you can stick in the headphones whilst you work out and go over any meetings, messages or work. This also works well for conference calls although you may not want to be doing anything to strenuous whilst on the phone. Pilates and yoga are good for this.

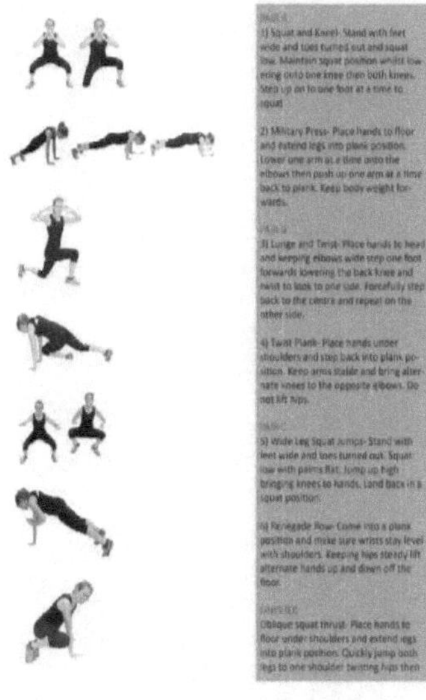

www.ingramcontent.com/pod-product-compliance
Lightning Source LLC
Chambersburg PA
CBHW020133180726

47992CB00022B/2931